I Once Was Fat but Now I'm Found:

Part 2 –Move Over Emotions, Make Room for Truth

by Laura Foote Fulford

I Once Was Fat but Now I'm Found: Part 2 – *Move Over Emotions, Make Room for Truth*

Written by Laura Foote Fulford

Copyright Laura Fulford 2019.

All rights reserved.

Published 2019.

ISBN: 9781093586046

Scripture quotations are from The ESV® Bible (The Holy Bible, English Standard Version®), copyright © 2001 by Crossway, a publishing ministry of Good News Publishers. Used by permission. All rights reserved.

"All things are lawful for me," but not all things are helpful. "All things are lawful for me," but I will not be dominated by anything."
- I Corinthians 6:12

Contents

Introduction	7
Chapter One: What is Fat?	13
Chapter Two: Calories, Metabolism, and Wishful Thinking	29
Chapter Three: If Dieting Doesn't Work, What Does?	49
Chapter Four: What Should I Eat (and why it's a useless question)?	69
Chapter Five: Exercise?	93
Final Word	107
Notes	111
About the Author	117

Introduction

The word "fat" is provocative. It evokes many emotions in people, including me. Even now, I associate the word with a host of awkward and painful memories.

One such memory takes me back to the years I worked in the banking world. I was in Chicago attending a big trade show. It was the Mortgage Banker Association's annual meeting and conference. It was the Super Bowl of mortgage banking. Legions of executives, men in power suits and perfectly dimpled ties and women adorned in Barbara Bush pearls and sensible shoes, would make the pilgrimage to Chicago.

The annual migration attracted thousands, like the March of the Penguins. They gathered to speak their unique banking language to each other. By using words like "yield spread premium" and "fungibility," the smart people enjoyed the status once reserved for the jocks and cheerleaders in high school.

Bankers prized special talents, such as doing long division in their heads. In this world, I had game. I "turned heads" with my mad spreadsheet skills. My high waist-to-hip ratio didn't seem to matter much in this world.

These were my people.

In this profession, I finally felt like "somebody." At times, I almost forgot that I was, in my own words, fat.

That crisp Chicago morning, the first day of the trade show, I was excited. I felt like I was going to the prom, only without the humiliation of not being asked. I got up early and went to the hotel's gym to rub elbows with all the execs, the ones wearing those little round glasses and sitting on recumbent bikes while reading the Wall Street Journal.

After my workout, I headed back to my room to ready myself. Shower—check. Hair—check. Makeup, pearls, control-top pantyhose, pumps—roger that. To top it off, I had a new red suit. Conservative, yet daring. It was a rare occasion when I *felt* like I looked good. I saw myself in the mirror, and I approved. My game-face was on.

I rode the elevator to the lobby and strode confidently out to catch a cab. I nodded to everyone, like Princess Diana on her way to dance with John Travolta. As the bellman opened the door to my taxi, I heard a female voice call from behind me, "Hey, would you mind sharing a cab?"

I glanced over my shoulder, and there she was. Time slowed down as if to offer everyone, including me, the chance to take it all in. She was nearly six feet tall, her long, brown hair was blowing in the wind, the collar was turned up on her white shirt, and she had a sassy, little scarf tied around her neck. Her long legs swept across the drive, draped in black pants cascading down into strappy high heel sandals. *Open toe shoes to a banking event?* I smirked to myself. *Not an insider*, I surmised. I tried to disguise my disdain for her exposed yet perfectly painted phalanges.

She cast a big, white-toothed smile to everyone who was staring at her, the "Glamazon" who looked like Cindy Crawford. I smiled at her, and we spoke pleasantly during the cab ride. In the back of my mind, a tiny, sarcastic, insecure gangster lurked, musing, "Ima cut her."

She confirmed what I suspected; she was not "one of us." She was a model hired to work at one of the trade show booths. I was further humiliated by how nice she was. I felt cheated not being able to find fault with her. Of course, in my mind, wouldn't we all be nice if we looked like Cindy Crawford?

Gazing at her perfect skin, hair, and features, my face felt rounder. My large feet felt bigger. I could feel the waistband of my control-tops rolling under the pressure of my belly fat. My game-face was crestfallen. She exited the cab and strolled off gracefully, turning heads and drawing attention as a beautiful woman does.

I let a few moments pass, then exited the cab behind the model, feeling my confidence crawl back inside me like a troll retreating under a bridge. I had entered the cab feeling like Princess Diana, and I left feeling like Shrek.

This story and many others in my life have risen and fallen on my longing for feeling unashamed only to be splashed with the cold water of my reality. I was fat. My fatness was the wrecking ball of every little thing I hoped would convince me I was worthy. Why did I think nothing else mattered but my weight? Why did I think my fat had so much power to confine me and steal my life from me? I was like the girl in the adipose bubble. But who was really keeping me there?

My perceptions were distorted. Yes, I was overweight, but my feelings about myself and my appearance were anything but objective, and anything but helpful.

In Part 2 of *I Once Was Fat, but Now I'm Found*, I'm inviting you to join me as we set aside our ever-wavering emotions. Why? Emotions obscure truth. Yes, they do need to be addressed. But first, let's set them aside and focus on what we can know for sure (and do) about losing fat.

What does God's design of our bodies teach us about losing weight, or more specifically, losing fat? The physical part of losing weight isn't so complicated or mysterious that we can't understand it and then use that understanding to our advantage. In algebra, when you know the constant, you can solve for the variable. When it comes to losing weight, it's helpful to know what we're dealing with physiologically so that we can solve for the other variables that make losing weight complex. The mental, emotional, and spiritual parts are not as straightforward. We'll address those in the next book, Part 3 of this series.

For now, you'll learn why fat, calories, metabolism, energy balance, basic nutrition, and exercise are the easy fundamentals you need to know to fight wisely and effectively in losing weight.

In Part 2, we'll visit questions such as:
- How does weight loss really work?
- What should I eat?
- How much do I need to exercise?

You may think you know the answers already, but when you consider the partial truths posing as weight loss wisdom, it's worth looking at truth you can really count on regarding the physiological process of losing weight.

Chapter One:
What is Fat?

Let the Battle Begin

Hardly anyone, upon hearing the word "fat" thinks immediately and only of a type of bodily tissue. For me, fat was many things. It was a never-ending jail sentence. It was the tormentor of my soul, the extinguisher of all the other redeeming qualities I probably had if only...

Rationally, of course, it wasn't true. But fat was all these other things to me for so long that it was difficult for me to see it for what it is and only for what it is.

Have you shared a similar misperception? If you're like me, maybe you've been fighting an emotional villain that lives large in your mind. For me, it not only lived there; that's where it claimed possession of my life.

As I was growing spiritually, I knew it was time to evict this mean, unwelcome, lying squatter.

Lies, when confronted with truth, become easier to evict.

Many lies had taken up residence around that three-letter word. Its real meaning had been crowded out. To reset my mind around the truth, I simply asked, "What is fat tissue?" and set out to replace the bad tenant with a good one.

Simply speaking, fat is a type of tissue among many other types, including skin, hair, muscle, bone, tendon, and cartilage. I don't freak out about my tendons, so why the frenzy over my fat tissue? I once saw on the Internet: "You are not fat. You have fat. You also have fingernails, but you are not fingernails." I don't know who said it originally, but if I ever find this person, I would like to hug her. It helped me put things into perspective.

In this chapter, we'll explore:

- What is fat tissue?
- What does it do?
- What are the health implications of having too much?

Then, in the following chapters, we'll cover what it takes, physiologically speaking, to lose fat tissue. Knowing these basics will help you separate fact from fiction when it comes to losing weight. Why is it so important to draw this distinction? If your emotions have influenced how you've pursued losing weight, then you need a steady "diet" of facts to keep you from falling prey to the seduction of "fast and easy." Don't let your emotions lead you to do things that sound promising but aren't possible.

Fat: God Made It

God, the architect of all of life, designed fat tissue. Like it or not, fat does what it does because God designed it to perform that way. Like all facets of His creation, fat tissue does all kinds of amazing things. When it doesn't do what we want it to do, it's reasonable to suspect we are doing something inconsistent with God's design. Therefore, we have three unavoidable truths to embrace:

- Fat tissue has been performing a variety of essential functions in the human body for as long as humans have existed and long before we were scientifically advanced enough to understand it.

- Fat tissue is inextricably connected to what we eat.

- We can and must learn how fat tissue operates so that we can stop making more of it and use up the extra we have accumulated.

We know more about fat now than we did when I was in college in the 80s. Back then, fat was thought to be an inactive tissue. Supposedly, it had no real job besides providing insulation, storing unused calories, and wearing out the inseams of my trousers.

Since then, we have found that fat is not just a gelatinous glob of unsightly body tissue. As tissue types go, fat is surprisingly busy. It's now known to be an endocrine organ.[1] That means, among other things, it makes hormones. It plays a role in fertility, energy availability, and other essential metabolic processes. Fat has many vital functions that benefit the human body. Even our brains need fat and are comprised of about 60% fat.[2]

Interestingly, however, we don't gain weight in our brains the way our bodies gain weight. In fact, the opposite occurs. As our body weight increases, our brains become smaller, and cognitive function declines.[3] The impact on brain functionality is only one among many health risks associated with carrying too much fat tissue. I had always been far more concerned about how my fat looked on me. In this culture, it's hard not to be. But the long-term risks of carrying too much fat are worth knowing. Then, you can decide whether it's worth a little effort now to avoid suffering later. As I age, I see the upside of avoiding as much suffering as I have the power to avoid. In light of that, please note:

- Obesity-related illnesses kill more of us than anything else.

- The longer we wait to do anything about it, the greater our exposure to serious health risks.

Let's look at a few more of the ways extra fat tissue can harm us.

The Health Risks of Excess Fat Tissue

When modern living conditions meet God's programming of the human body to survive, what happens? An obesity epidemic. In America, we have an abundance of food and not much need to move. Our lives are dramatically different from our ancestors. The chances are that the males in your family are not out hunting wooly mammoths to feed your young. Domino's Pizza makes such activities unnecessary.

Is it progress or tragedy that one can "hunt" in a video game sitting mostly motionless and waiting for the pizza to arrive on the doorstep?

Our living conditions make it not only easy but likely that we'll accumulate too much fat tissue and set us on course for a wide variety of health problems. When fat grows past a certain point on your body, it turns mean and wants to kill you–albeit, usually slowly.

According to Dr. David L. Katz, Director of the Yale Prevention Research Center, "The four leading causes of death among adults in America are heart disease, cancer, stroke, and diabetes. Obesity is on the causal pathway to every one of those."[4] Excess fat tissue is the primary accomplice in the four deadliest of all American diseases. With 2 of every 3 Americans either overweight or obese, the chances are good that you or someone you know is currently at risk. Isn't it ironic that the way Americans live and eat is also the way most of us die?

The more we accumulate fat tissue, the greater its impact on us. Because the accumulation happens so gradually, most don't realize how extensively their health is compromised until a severe event occurs, such as a heart attack or a stroke.

Consider the following list of diseases and warning signs that go hand in hand with carrying too much fat tissue. Do any of these affect you currently? [5]

- Coronary heart disease
- High blood pressure
- Stroke
- High cholesterol and abnormal blood fats
- Fatigue
- Shortness of breath (obesity hypoventilation syndrome)
- Type 2 diabetes or pre-diabetes diagnosis
- Metabolic syndrome
- Cancer
- Osteoarthritis
- Chronic pain
- Inflammation
- Reproductive problems
- Gallstones
- Non-alcoholic fatty liver disease
- Sleep apnea

Even children are being affected by many of these "adult" illnesses, such as non-alcoholic fatty liver disease. When overweight children grow into overweight adults, they can pass unexpected consequences to their children. Research shows that excessive fat tissue in men affects male fertility, sperm function, and the health of their children. "Data from animal models implicate the nutritional status of the father as setting the developmental trajectory of resultant offspring. Both male and female offspring born to fathers with sub-optimal nutrition have a constellation of metabolic and reproductive health pathologies."[6] Translation: the more fat tissue the father of a child carries, the more health issues are passed to the child. As each generation's kids have kids, we are witnessing more obesity and poorer health being passed down.

Carrying extra weight is risky. *Where* we carry it matters in assessing the extent of the risk.

Apples and Pears

I am an apple-shaped girl. I have friends who are pear-shaped. When I was heavier, my fat accumulated around my waist, squished up into my armpits, and "mooshed" into my upper arms. Pears tend to carry extra weight below the waist in the hips, thighs, and "hindquarters." As fat distribution goes, the pears have a slight advantage. Even so, any body type, and even thin-looking people, can accumulate the more dangerous type of fat. It's important to pay attention to where it is.

There are two types of fat, distinguished by where they sit. The fat that is under the skin but outside of the abdominal wall is called subcutaneous fat. The fat that grows inside the abdominal cavity is called visceral fat. [4] Subcutaneous is the less-concerning of the two. What makes visceral fat more dangerous? Three things, primarily: organ crowding, toxic secretions, and appetite deregulation.

Fat Gone Wild

When fat tissue grows inside the abdominal cavity, it crowds the stomach, liver, intestines, kidneys, lungs, and diaphragm. It's not a friendly neighbor. It not only sidles up too closely, but it also has toxic parties. It's a bit like a bad chemistry experiment happening inside your abdomen.

Recall, as stated earlier, that fat tissue behaves like an endocrine organ. It's the endocrine or hormonal activity that makes secretions inside the abdominal cavity. These secretions from fat tissue are poisonous. "Excess visceral fat is linked to Type 2 Diabetes, insulin resistance, a host of inflammatory illnesses and other gravely serious diseases." [7] Those other diseases include heart disease, high blood pressure, stroke, and some cancers. [5] The secretions of fat tissue also make their way into the liver and contribute to non-alcoholic fatty liver disease, or NAFLD. Recall NAFLD is one of the diseases appearing in younger and younger children.

As if the stress on your organs wasn't concerning enough, fat tissue also messes with your appetite. Normally, our fat tissue's beneficial activities would include appetite regulation and calling on fat to be used for energy. But excess fat tissue causes the hormones related to normal fat metabolism–leptin, ghrelin, insulin, resistin, and adiponectin—to go awry. [8] These are the main hormones involved in appetite regulation, fat storage, and fat usage.

At a healthy weight, the human body gives us normal hunger and fullness signals, stable blood sugar, and normal fat storage functionality. But as fat tissue increases, it impairs normal function. Then, what happens? We lose normal hunger and fullness awareness. Then, we grow even more likely to overeat and keep accumulating fat.

I used to think my increasing ability to gain weight was in my head. But there are physiological reasons why the more weight we gain, the more weight we are likely to gain. All those hormones involved in regulating appetite, blood sugar, and fat storage become confused and stop doing what they are supposed to do. If you ever have a hard time telling the difference between when you are "hungry" or "full," and if you find that you gain weight more and more readily, you may be experiencing the effects of your hunger and satisfaction hormones going awry.

How does one turn the tide of weight gain and get a handle on fat tissue gone wild? We'll continue to pursue the steps we can take to turn the tide.

Reflections

If wanting to be thin burned calories, I'd have turned into vapor back in the early 70s. My emotions clouded my perceptions and made losing weight all but impossible. How I made decisions was based on how I felt rather than what was factual. I knew the facts, but I avoided them for as long as I could. I held out for answers that sounded miraculous and swept me up into hope and inspiration, while requiring very little of me in the process.

For me, learning the facts wasn't a "Eureka" moment that snapped me onto the right path. Honestly, hardly anyone is motivated to lose weight simply by learning the facts or even the health risks. Nevertheless, the facts will help you in several important ways:

- They will counterbalance the emotions that get in your way.

- They will help you compare the cost to your life and health and the benefit of making progressive changes.

In this chapter, we've started building your arsenal of weapons to confront your uncooperative the emotions. You can avoid another emotionally driven rededication to a "miracle" weight loss program. Let's map out your next steps based on a foundation of facts about the way your body works when it comes to fat tissue–whether storing it or using it.

As we touch on some of the basic physical and physiological inner workings of losing fat tissue, keep in mind that we are working our way through layers of the battle, starting with the body and working our way inward. It helps to keep the practical side of the journey as straightforward as possible.

Questions

Take your time with these questions. I recommend you write out your answers. You can also print these questions from Stop Dieting for Life (https://stopdietingforlife.com/).

1. What emotions have you wrestled with when it comes to your weight?

2. Can you recall times when you have embarked on a weight loss program based on strong emotions? Describe them.

3. How do you feel about your weight right now?

4. What would it be like if the negative emotions about your weight were gone?

Read Psalm 139: 1-18.

O LORD, you have searched me and known me!
² You know when I sit down and when I rise up;

you discern my thoughts from afar.
³ You search out my path and my lying down
  and are acquainted with all my ways.
⁴ Even before a word is on my tongue,
  behold, O Lord, you know it altogether.
⁵ You hem me in, behind and before,
  and lay your hand upon me.
⁶ Such knowledge is too wonderful for me;
  it is high; I cannot attain it.
⁷ Where shall I go from your Spirit?
  Or where shall I flee from your presence?
⁸ If I ascend to heaven, you are there!
  If I make my bed in Sheol, you are there!
⁹ If I take the wings of the morning
  and dwell in the uttermost parts of the sea,
¹⁰ even there your hand shall lead me,
  and your right hand shall hold me.
¹¹ If I say, "Surely the darkness shall cover me,
  and the light about me be night,"
¹² even the darkness is not dark to you;
  the night is bright as the day,
  for darkness is as light with you.
¹³ For you formed my inward parts;
  you knitted me together in my mother's womb.
¹⁴ I praise you, for I am fearfully and wonderfully made.
Wonderful are your works;
  my soul knows it very well.
¹⁵ My frame was not hidden from you,

when I was being made in secret,
    intricately woven in the depths of the earth.
16 Your eyes saw my unformed substance;
in your book were written, every one of them,
    the days that were formed for me,
    when as yet there was none of them.
17 How precious to me are your thoughts, O God!
    How vast is the sum of them!
18 If I would count them, they are more than the sand.
    I awake, and I am still with you.

5. How well does the Lord know David? Describe what David says the Lord knows about him.

6. Why do you think David thought the Lord's work is so wonderful?

7. What attributes of the human body cause you to marvel at God's work?

8. Write a prayer of thanks to the Lord for specific attributes of your living body (for instance, eyes that see, ears that hear, lungs that breathe, a heart that beats, and a brain that thinks, reacts, and regulates...)

Chapter Two:
Calories, Metabolism, and Wishful Thinking

Do calories matter? Can I speed up my metabolism? These are common questions. If I had any power over the universe, I'd find the knobs that control those two settings. While I was in that cosmic control room, I'd also be tempted to give gravity a nudge so that I would weigh only 110 pounds.

Unfortunately, these things are out of reach for mortals. Why, then, are we bombarded by advertising claims like these?

- Never count *calories* again!
- "Rev up" your *metabolism*!
- Lose 30 pounds in 30 days!
- Burn fat while you sleep!

I'll tell you why. Because these are dog whistles that will bring every dieter running with hopes high and wallets open.

I confess that those kinds of ads worked on me, even when I knew they were nonsense. I wanted what they were selling so badly, I was willing to try any product *just in case* it did what the advertiser claimed.

Because I have fallen for so many false claims out of my last-ditch desperation, I feel duty-bound to share what you can really expect when it comes to calories and metabolism. You might still long for a miracle, but at least you'll know it's not coming and perhaps save yourself a few dollars in the process.

Be comforted; you're about to add real weapons to your weight loss arsenal. When you know why calories matter and to what extent you can successfully manipulate the speed of your metabolism, you'll have the stepping stones for the next chapter, where you'll learn what's involved in losing fat tissue.

Confessions of a Fat Fitness Professional

After college, I worked in a fitness facility that was part of a yacht club. Some of the patrons reminded me of the rich couple on *Gilligan's Island*, Thurston Howell III and his wife, Lovey. Amidst my duties of personal training, teaching classes, and learning boating lingo, I also exercised feverishly, taking full advantage of all the fitness equipment at my disposal. I was very fit. I could keep up with the thinnest of the thin and strongest of the strong.

Despite the exercise, I remained 30-40 pounds overweight. It puzzled me, especially considering I ate almost nothing all day. *Almost* nothing. How could I still be overweight?

This was during the 1980s when everyone believed dietary fat was the enemy. Fat-free foods were the rage. Pasta was king. Bagels were the Boss of breadstuffs.

Following the trend, my "weight management" strategy was to eat little or no fat. After eating as little as possible during the day, I went home to a large, low-fat, high-carb dinner. I was not losing weight. In fact, I was gaining weight. Every effort I made was working against me. My exercise, my low-fat/high-carb eating, and this other habit I pretended not to notice.

Each workday, while I was "woman-handling" my hunger pangs, refusing to feed them breakfast or lunch, I appeased my growling tummy with a bite here and there of this innocent-looking candy. Stationed throughout the fitness center were colorful little dishes of candy-coated mints. Every time I passed by a dish, I would eat a small handful of those mints. By the end of each day, those little mints I wasn't counting as "food" still added up. When I did the math, it was close to 1,000 calories. Those 1,000 extra calories were over and above what I would eat for dinner when I arrived home ravenous.

While I was eating "almost nothing" all day, I failed to consider those extra calories of candy I ate mindlessly, a little at a time. The candy did nothing to make me feel the slightest bit full or satisfied. I constantly felt hungry, which made it easy to trick myself into thinking I was "starving myself" and truly "watching what I ate." Of course, I was deceiving myself. I was sure I had some mysterious metabolic malady, with all this working out and starving I was doing.

Mystery solved. No, my metabolism wasn't slow. I wasn't just big-boned or "solid." I was eating too many calories every day, not to mention the wrong kind. All the calories I consumed but didn't count molded me into an overweight fitness professional. My body simply responded to what I fed it—more calories than it needed every day. Not to mention, the wrong kind, a topic we'll touch on later.

Calories - Who Cares?

Why should anyone care about calories? What exactly is a calorie anyway?

The scientist's definition of the kind of calories we eat goes like this: the amount of heat needed to raise the temperature of one liter of water by one degree Celsius.[9] That's neither helpful nor interesting. Yet as soon as losing fat tissue becomes a concern, calories become vital to the conversation. I'm not saying calories are the whole conversation, but I am saying they cannot be excluded. Calories will always be relevant, along with the other relevant variables that make losing weight a bit of a puzzle.

"Calorie" is the name humans gave to something God made: energy. In nutrition circles, calories refer to the amount of energy stored in food.

Our bodies also have energy mini-storage units. We have some short-term storage units in our muscles, and some long-term storage units called fat cells. For the moment, let's focus on the long-term storage units, our fat cells.

Here is where the caramel meets the nougat. The extra calories we eat and don't burn have to go somewhere. There's nowhere else for them to go but to get added to the excess stored energy (fat) on our bodies. So, do extra calories matter? Yes.

If science makes your head hurt, place one hand on your cerebral cortex for about 10 seconds. I'm about to tell you the "science-y" reason calories will *always* matter.

Do you remember the *Law of Conservation of Energy* from a high school or college science class? Here's the summary: energy cannot be created or destroyed. Neither you nor I can "make" energy, nor can we snap our fingers and eliminate energy that already exists. Only God has that kind of power.

For us, this is an inconvenient truth about losing weight. All the energy (calories) we eat must go somewhere. We will use some of the energy in our bodily activities. But when we eat excess calories that are not used up in activity, we will store the excess as fat. There is no other possibility for them. Extra calories remain in our fat cells until we use them.

Calories will always matter. Can we use this to our advantage? Most definitely.

How does your body know when it has had too many calories and begins to store them? Is it possible for you to know when that starts happening and prevent it?

Your Metabolic Rate: The Father's Daily Allowance

Another inescapable weight loss truth is this: our bodies burn a *limited* number of calories each day. Your *metabolic rate* represents the speed of your metabolism. Because each 24-hour period ends, and during that time you have burned a finite number of calories, you do, indeed, have a calorie limit. Consider this limit your calorie allowance. If you exceed your allowance, you'll store the extra calories.

Your *metabolism* is like your body's engine. Your engine and its parts perform all the inner functions and processes that keep you alive. Your organ function, growth, repair, and many other processes all comprise your metabolism. These are continuously running bodily processes require energy and, thus, burn calories. For example, brain activity alone uses about 20% of the calories we burn overall. Yes, that three-pound blob of pudding-like substance in your skull uses about one-fifth of the calories you burn every day.[10] The rest of your body runs on the other four-fifths. The brain and body activities that keep you alive comprise your metabolism. The number of calories your body uses in just these processes (not including your activity) every 24 hours is your basal metabolic rate.

Your body burns a finite number of calories in every 24-hour cycle. Suppose the number was 1,800 calories. This means if you ate 1,800 calories that day, you would have matched your calorie needs. Imagine 1,800 is the tipping point. Over 1,800, you've eaten more calories than you burned and accumulated some extra energy. Under 1,800, you've created a demand for energy stored in your body.

The reason I want you to grasp this tipping point idea is to give you a handy navigational tool. How can you use this to your advantage when it comes to managing your weight?

Tipping Over?

What happens when you spend more money than you have? The bank notifies you. What happens when you eat more calories than you burn? The scale notifies you. In both cases, you become aware after the fact that you have crossed a tipping point to the side you don't want to be on.

Here is the perfect storm for exceeding your calorie tipping point:

1. Not knowing how many calories you burn in a day.

2. Not knowing how many calories you eat in a day.

3. Eating the standard American diet and not giving calories any thought.

If any of these three points are true of you, then it's likely you are consuming too many calories for your body, even if you believe you're eating healthy. Plainly speaking, the extra calories you eat cause your body to accumulate more fat tissue and for your weight to increase.

Neglecting to get a grip on your calorie inputs and outputs is like spending money without checking your bank account. Overspending gets you into financial trouble. Isn't overeating similar?

So, how can you take cover from the perfect calorie storm and tip your body into using fat rather than storing fat?

1. Learn what your metabolic rate is.
2. Monitor how many calories you eat in a day.
3. Adjust your calorie intake to less than your calorie expenditure

Admittedly, measuring your metabolic rate is an inexact science, as you'll see below, but that's okay. Again, the point of doing this is not precision but control. You can effectively manage your body's use and storage of fat tissue. If there was ever a "secret" to success, practically speaking, this is it. Why? Monitoring your calories places you in control over the inputs and outputs that tell your body to store fat or use stored fat.

Are there other factors that affect the outcome? Yes. All I'm doing here is pointing to one that gives you the most control and measurability.

Let's look at how to determine the calories your body burns in a day.

How to Determine Your Metabolic Rate

Your metabolic rate is affected by your gender, height, weight, and age. Still other factors come into play, which explains why two people of the same, gender, height, weight and age may still have different metabolic rates. That said, let's estimate yours.

It helps to know two different metabolism measures. One is like your idle speed, and the other is like your cruising speed.

Your idle speed, or **resting metabolic rate** (RMR), is the number of calories your body uses at rest. You may also hear it referred to as the Basal Metabolic Rate (BMR).[11] For our purposes, your RMR is the amount of energy needed to keep your body going when you lie at rest.

The second measure is your **daily metabolic rate**. This "cruising speed" number is simply the additional calories you burn in performing activity each day above your BMR. In a typical 24 hours, you sleep part of it and are active during the other part. Your body functions at the resting rate during sleeping hours and increases after you get up and go. The total number of calories you burn during a 24-hour cycle is your Daily Metabolic Rate. Think of it like this:

Your sleeping calories + the calories burned in your waking hours = Your Daily Rate

Think of your daily rate as the *tipping point* I mentioned earlier, the fulcrum that sits between storing extra calories as fat and burning stored calories as fuel.

- If calories eaten = calories burned, your weight would stay the same.

- If calories eaten > calories burned, your body stores the extra.

- If calories eaten < calories burned, your body will draw on stored calories.

Your body has a real teetering point where fat tissue is either accumulated or is used. As you would guess, your teetering point is a little higher on your more active days and lower on less active days. This is an oversimplification of a complex process, BUT don't miss this. I'll be showing you how it can make a big difference in your weight loss success.

3 Ways to Determine Your Metabolic Rate

Your metabolic rate can be determined in three different ways, which vary in accuracy and accessibility.

- **Direct Calorimetry:** This is the most *accurate* way to measure your metabolism, but the equipment for the procedure is hard to come by.

- **Indirect Calorimetry:** Often available in portable and hand-held devices, indirect calorimeters estimate your metabolic rate by analyzing the exchange of oxygen and carbon dioxide as you breathe into the device for a short period of time. These are accurate if used correctly. They are also much more accessible.

- **Calculation:** Calculations provide an estimate of your rate based on your height, age, and weight. It is the least accurate of these three ways, but it's easy, readily accessible, and it gets the job done.

The ease and accessibility of calculating your metabolic rate offer you something powerful and immediate: a tool you can use right now to manage your weight. The alternative is eating, guessing, and hoping for the best.

How well has eating, guessing, and hoping worked for you in the past? For me, it only allowed me to continue to deceive myself about what I was eating and how much.

Doing the Calculation

Google will lead to many sites to estimate your metabolic rate. You can also visit the one on my website, StopDietingForLife.com and use the metabolic rate calculator provided on the *Resources* page. You'll also find that MyFitnessPal can help you determine your rate and the number of calories it recommends you eat in a given day.

Americans are bad at the calorie-guessing game. How do I know? The worsening obesity epidemic proves it. In our processed food-loving culture, it is ridiculously easy to eat more calories than our bodies need.

Knowing your metabolic rate gives you a tremendous advantage. Used correctly, it can help you stop gaining and start losing weight.

Now that you know your tipping point, we can take it a step further in the next chapter when we talk about energy balance. Before we leave the topic of metabolism, though, let's touch briefly on speed.

Metabolism: The Need for Speed

Doesn't everyone who struggles with weight wish for a faster metabolism? Unfortunately, your personal "idle speed" is not particularly adjustable. As mentioned earlier, your metabolism is comprised of many complex and inter-related bodily processes that keep you alive. Considering the complexity of all the intricately interwoven bodily systems involved, and our myopic desire to lose weight, the Lord was wise and merciful to keep this particular "dial" well-hidden from us.

The phrase "rev up" (when it precedes the word metabolism) has always bothered me. Perhaps because it is a hollow tease I fell for too many times. The two most common methods promoted to boost metabolism are supplements and building muscle mass. I've tried both, even knowing better.

Supplements and Foods

It is true that some foods and supplements have a *mild* "thermogenic" or calorie burning effect. They may speed up metabolism *slightly*—as in by a few calories. The actual effect is insufficient to warrant eating an extra half-cup of blueberries, much less the all-you-can-eat blank check our minds might conjure up. I tried nearly every supplement in existence until around 2005. Some of the ones I tried through the years were found to be risky and have since been taken off the market.

Products containing Green Coffee Bean Extract, Hoodia, Garcinia Cambogia, Raspberry Ketones, and others have all had their share of publicity. Why do we purchase these things? We hope they will make a significant difference. My experience is this:

- They gave me false hope that I could eat more or would lose weight faster or both.

- They delivered no noticeable benefit–no weight loss, no appetite suppression, nothing.

- Some of them *revved up* my irritability and anxiety but not my metabolism.

- Taking them delayed me from taking responsibility and real action.

- When they failed, I was left more discouraged than when I started.

When it comes to supplements or products that promise to speed up your metabolism, my recommendation is to avoid them. Many products have side effects, and none of them will compensate for exceeding your daily calorie limit. You will accomplish much more knowing the truth about your body, and you won't need the products.

"Packing On" Muscle

You have probably heard that having more muscle increases your metabolism. It does. But how much speed can you count on from "packing on lean muscle?" Again, let's apply a dose of realism. There are two caveats to consider: 1) how much the extra muscle burns and 2) what it takes to gain even one pound of muscle.

For years, claims circulated that every pound of muscle we gain burns 50 extra calories per day. For example, three pounds of newly packed-on muscle would buy you an additional 150 calories per day. Unfortunately, the actual number is closer to 6-10 calories per pound of muscle.[12] So, those three extra pounds of sinewy firmness will give you an extra 18-30 calorie boost in your daily metabolic rate. No doubt, building muscle has benefits, but *revving* your metabolic rate overstates the effect.

Also, women aren't naturally able to put on more than a few pounds of muscle mass over a long period of time. To put on three pounds of muscle might require 3-6 months of hard work. Make no mistake, the health benefits of building muscle are great and worth the effort, especially if you enjoy the workouts. The traps to avoid, though, are:

- Don't chase working out just to move the scale faster.

- Be careful not to assume a plateau or even weight gain is because you are gaining muscle.

In both cases, monitoring your calories can explain what the scale is doing.

By clarifying what you can and can't accomplish to change your idle speed, I hope to point you back to the most realistic and effective place to devote your attention and effort when it comes to managing your weight: how much you eat, as well as the quality of the food you eat. We will dive deeper into quality and food choices in Chapter Four.

Reflections

On my way to the truth about my weight problem, I had to chip away at years of experimenting with ways to lose weight faster and easier. I did everything to avoid facing how much I was eating.

Have you been excited about a fast weight loss promise or enticed to think a pill will help you lose weight while you sleep? Have you been seduced by compelling "before and after" photos? Chasing those promises may be more harmful than helpful. They are unworthy of your hope.

How does God see your situation? Offer your hope to the One who made you. He has already given us the truth. He can and will help us change our relationship with food. Knowing the truth about our bodies is an important part of the puzzle and a step in the direction of real change.

Rest in knowing that God designed our bodies. The more we know about His plan, the better we can align ourselves with His intentions. The more we grow to love Him, the more delightful it becomes to align ourselves with Him.

Questions
Read Colossians 2:8.

See to it that no one takes you captive by philosophy and empty deceit, according to human tradition, according to the elemental spirits of the world, and not according to Christ.

1. How would you describe "human traditions" of the culture we live in, especially related to weight and appearance? How does this cultural perspective conflict with what is true from God's Word?

2. When you think about losing weight, to what extent do you wish for something to make it fast and easy?

3. What kinds of things have you tried because you believed they would be fast and/or easy?

4. When it comes to losing weight, what uncomfortable things would you avoid doing if you could?

5. When you write out the things that make you uncomfortable, ask yourself why. Pray about each one.

The most uncomfortable things for me were 1) acknowledging how much I was really eating and 2) acknowledging that I was eating for reasons that had little to do with satisfying hunger or nourishing my body. I was an emotional eater and often sought food the way someone might seek alcohol or drugs.

These are issues we'll explore further in the next book, Part 3. For now, let's continue to lay a foundation of facts about our bodies. I simply wanted you to know that we'll be talking about the emotions that make this process difficult.

Chapter Three:
If Dieting Doesn't Work, What Does?

Tracing our steps, in Chapter One, we exposed fat tissue's cantankerous side, and why having less of it will benefit us. In Chapter Two, we covered calories and metabolism. These point us to a tipping point where our bodies could begin to use our stored fat tissue if pressed to do so. The existence of a real calorie tipping point tees up the next question perfectly: How do we tip ourselves over to the fat burning side of the equation?

Our bodies are infinitely complex, and how fat is used and stored is no exception. The good news is that we don't need to fully understand or even articulate the complexity to accomplish what we desire: losing weight, specifically in the form of fat tissue. If you are tired of floundering and getting nowhere, then gird up your mind; this is for you.

As we discussed, it is *inescapable* that calories play a role in managing our weight. Not only a role but a starring role. We've established that ignoring calories is to ignore the one handle you can grab to get control over the otherwise maddeningly elusive process of trying to manage your weight.

It's true that to burn stored fat, you must do one thing over and over: burn more calories than you eat. It sounds so easy. But we already know it's tricky. It's akin to suggesting that golf is easy; all you must do is get that little ball in the hole 18 times. But if you have ever played golf, you know there's a tad more to it than that.

Just as golfing is more than riding the links with cart and clubs, losing fat is more than signing up and weighing in. Your "sleeves up" participation is required.

You *can* learn how to lose fat. It will require attention, intention, patience, knowledge, and practice. Just as in golf, not many people get good at it unless they practice consistently and in the right way.

Consider this: compare all the effort you've made in your life to lose weight vs. the results you achieved with your effort. How do they compare? Would you like to even the score?

In this chapter, you'll learn the best way to match the effort you make to lose weight with the outcome of losing fat tissue. There may be countless ways to the green, but skilled golfers get the ball in the hole with the fewest strokes. Likewise, make your effort count.

How Tracking Calories Beats Dieting

Many popular diet programs claim that if you eat as prescribed, you will lose weight and won't need to track calories. That may be true. But when you choose that route for losing weight, it's important to be aware of what you are giving up for the "ease" of having your eating decisions mapped out for you by someone else.

Imagine you are a passenger being driven along an unfamiliar route and dropped off at an equally unfamiliar destination. How would you find your way there the next time? How would you find your way around if you got there?

You don't learn much when you are the passenger rather than the driver. Dieting is like that. It might get you there, but it won't teach you how to get there on your own, much less, how to stay there. Is that a trade-off you want to make? For the ease of the ride in the short-run, you weaken yourself in the long-run. You gave up learning how to navigate your own way.

The more a diet program does the thinking for you, the less prepared you'll be to navigate the normal curves of life when you no longer follow the diet. Diets end for many reasons:

- You plateau or start gaining weight again.

- You are interrupted by something unexpected.

- You get sick of the food.

- It's too much trouble to follow the plan.

- You deviate from the plan and then, derail yourself because you feel like you "blew it."

- You get impatient and start to improvise when progress slows down

Any number of things can interrupt a good streak of "diet-compliant eating." Then, once interrupted, before you can say Toaster Strudel, the weight you lost comes back. Then, what? Most people slide back into the decisions that govern their eating habits between diets. The essential lessons diets don't teach you include:

- What do I do when I plateau?

- What do I do when I am sick of the plan?

- How do I keep the weight off?

- How do I know what to eat when the food that is "on the diet" isn't available?

- How do I get back on track when I mess up for a few days? Or weeks?

- How do I find my motivation again when I give up and am too frustrated to care?

Diets don't teach you how to do any of these things. When all you learn is "you eat the food, you lose the weight," as one popular program proclaims, you aren't left with much to work with when you are sick of the food and gaining the weight back.

What's not being said in the flashy commercials? Most people don't reach their goals, they don't lose nearly as much weight as the program suggests, and most, by far, gain the weight back.

In a study published in the *Journal of the American Medical Association*, only 50-65% of participants stuck with popular diet programs, and they still only averaged small losses of between 2 and 3.5 pounds.[13] The claims of diet programs do not prove themselves in scientific studies, especially when you look at long-term results.

All programs that treat weight as *the problem* to be solved and dieting as *the solution* are doomed to fail. As we progress, it will become increasingly clear that your weight is not the problem; it's a symptom. Likewise, dieting is not the answer; it's a Band-Aid.

Diets fall short of teaching you how to live and manage your weight. Most of all, diets don't address the root cause of the problem. (Again, this is the topic of Part 3 of this series)

To be clear, tracking our food intake is just part of the solution. But its clear advantages over dieting are as follows:

- The only way to lose fat is to use it. Tracking your calories lets you manage achieving and sustaining a calorie deficit day by day.

- Tracking your calories helps you interpret what's happening on the scale. It gives you the data you need to adjust as you go, keeping you in control of your results.

In a nutshell, tracking places you in the driver's seat, whereas dieting places you in the passenger seat.

I admit, the idea of not dealing with calories is enticing. It's as enticing as having a credit card with no limit, or a blank check from a rich uncle's bank account.

Here are a few more things to consider if you'd like to be in the driver's seat when it comes to your weight loss. With these guidelines, you'll be free to mold a plan you like and don't mind following long-term.

Calories...Who's Counting?

If you want to be the belle of the weight loss ball, just proclaim, "no calorie-counting ever!" Many weight loss companies and gurus scoff at the idea of "counting" calories. It's popular to promise what people want to hear. Who really wants to think about calories? But what's the trade-off?

I *could* design a food plan for you, telling you exactly what to eat. To do that for you, I would have to make sure it is calorie controlled, or guess what? You won't lose weight. So, even if you didn't count the calories, I did it for you.

Newsflash: Whether you count your calories or not, your body does. If you are doing someone else's plan, then they "counted" them for you when they constructed the plan.

If you are losing weight, regardless of the program, your body is experiencing a calorie deficit. If you begin gaining weight on that program, it's because you are exceeding your body's calorie limit.

Calories will always matter when it comes to managing weight.

Here's the thing: We have a built-in tendency to nibble our way right past our calorie boundaries, even when eating healthy. My appetite doesn't magically turn off as soon as I reach the calories I need for the day.

I cannot *feel* my metabolic tipping point. I can't detect my fat cells opening to welcome my extra calories. Fullness doesn't tell you. I might feel full after eating a big bowl of spinach or a big bowl of ice cream. But the two bowlfuls could be a distinction of hundreds of calories.

Have you ever been able to determine how many calories you ate based on how full you felt? That's like determining how much money you have in your bank account by how many checks you have left. One is not a reliable measure of the other.

Left to my natural appetite, I'll eat far more calories than I need. I like food, and even healthy food tastes good to me—good enough to overeat. I can gain weight month over month and year over year eating healthy food when I don't track my calories.

The point? Even with the healthiest of health foods, we cannot allow ourselves a blank check to eat all we want. Health gurus will throw around phrases like "plenty of..." People like me do not need to hear phrases like that, especially in the same sentence as words like avocado, cashews, almond butter, and roasted chickpeas.

Are good calories magically different than bad calories? Do healthy and unhealthy calories act differently once you have passed your daily calorie limit? No, those "healthy" calories will still be stored as fat too. Not to mention, how often do your extra calories come from celery? Probably never. Why? Because we naturally prefer higher-calorie foods, even the healthy ones.

Quality and Equality: How Do Calories Matter?

One prevalent argument I frequently hear against counting calories is that not all calories are "created equal." I know what they mean, but first, let's be technically accurate.

The truth is that 100 calories are 100 calories whether they come from broccoli, peanut butter, or Twinkies. Just as an inch is an inch, a calorie is a calorie. But an inch of a rubber band is different from an inch of a diamond tennis bracelet.

The quality of your calories does vary from food to food. Calories from processed foods are more problematic than whole foods that occur in nature. Processed foods are higher in calorie density, lower in absorbable nutrients, and often contain ingredients that are unhealthy if consumed regularly. Could I eat 1,200-1,400 calories of chocolate chip cookies a day and lose weight? Technically, yes. A study published in the *New England Journal of Medicine* concluded, "Reduced-calorie diets result in clinically meaningful weight loss regardless of which macronutrients they emphasize."[14] You may recall the Twinkie Diet, based on this proven premise.

The problem with the Twinkie Diet or any diet built around low-quality calories is not the number of calories themselves. Your body doesn't just need calories; it needs nutrients to be healthy. In the next chapter, we will discuss further why *what* we choose to eat is as important as *limiting how much* we eat. Both will always matter because of the way God designed our bodies; we need energy *and* nutrients.

Remember, no person, process, pill, or program can make the Law of Conservation of Energy untrue. So, I'll conclude this section with these two recommendations:

1) Track your food/calorie intake daily using an app like MyFitnessPal

2) Eat foods that God made and progressively eliminate processed foods from your routine food choices.

Tracking calories daily removes the mystery of how much I'm eating. It also prevents me from lying to myself that I am "dieting" when, in fact, I'm gaining weight from eating too many calories. More than anything now, I aim to honor my God-given allowance, by the limits He designed into my body.

What's Your Number?

Now that we have established the conditions for using our stored fat, the next question is this: Can we facilitate the process? And the answer is yes.

When does your body use its stored fat? When it runs out of other fuel. The easiest fuel for your body to use comes from the food you ate most recently, not from your stored fat. If you have eaten just enough or more than enough to fuel your body's activity, it won't need to disturb the fat in storage. But if losing fat tissue is your aim, then those fat stores must be disturbed and gradually depleted. It takes a while to accomplish this, and for good reason. God designed the human body to be efficient and adaptable for survival.

What must you do to make the mystical transition into fat burning?

The Art and Science of Fat Loss

The math that helps us estimate fat loss is just that, an estimate. Keep in mind, though, that we are giving ourselves a steering wheel and guardrails, not doing laser surgery.

This may be familiar to you. But if you haven't put it into practice yet, it's worth reviewing.

Each pound of fat holds roughly 3,500 calories of stored energy. So, to lose about one pound of stored fat, we must work through those 3,500 (or so) calories by putting our bodies in the place of needing to use them. Then, we must continue working our way through each successive pound until we find ourselves at the healthier weight of our choosing. Granted, the process is not as precise as the math would imply (for a variety of reasons), but it is still an effective way to manage your progress.

Apps like MyFitnessPal will help you determine a reasonable calorie target for each day to establish the deficit. You may want to aim for *averaging* this amount. For instance, if I am aiming to eat 1,500 calories per day, I would want to make sure that by the end of the week, I had *averaged* 1,500 calories. I might eat 1,750 on one day and 1,250 on another day to compensate.

Our Built-In Limitations to Fast Weight Loss

Many factors beyond our control determine how fast we lose weight. Even so, proactively managing your calories gives you more control than any other tool to manage an otherwise unpredictable and often frustrating process.

We can't rush losing weight very much. Our bodies won't let us. There are many reasons why about losing 1 pound (or less) each week is a reasonable goal. You can also expect the pace to start off fast but then, slow down more and more as you get closer to your target weight range.

Why is it wise to avoid fast weight loss? It requires extreme measures over a long period of time. Not only is it difficult to sustain such measures, but your body will begin working against you. I used to aim for losing two pounds per week. This meant creating a 1,000-calorie deficit every day. To do that, I either had to exercise like a mad dog or cut way (*way*) back on calories, or both. I generally tried to do it mostly with exercise.

Either way, our bodies are adaptable and will adjust to become more "efficient." As noted in an article published by Precision Nutrition, "Metabolic adaptation is a natural defense mechanism against starvation. When you're dieting, at a certain point, your body will send up a red flag. *Starvation alert! There's not enough food to go around! Hold onto the fat reserves!* At that point, your RMR slows."[15]

If you eat 500 calories per day consistently, your body will adjust to its lower fuel level. If you exercise feverishly, your body will adapt and become more efficient, burning fewer calories with the same exercise. You might be hoping for a Mac truck metabolism, but your actions may be turning your body into a Prius. Don't let your impatience lead you into these mistakes.

It might be *possible* to create a 1,000-calorie deficit for a day here and there, but over the long-run, it is a self-defeating strategy. For most people, the effort is too hard, and both results and motivation will wane.

Our bodies won't cooperate with extreme demands for weight loss. God designed our bodies to adjust to the demands we place on them. If you give your body less food and ask it to work harder, it will accommodate the shortage by slowing its metabolism to ensure its survival. The body's built-in instinct to preserve itself and survive was essential in less modern times, but today, it has spoiled many a bathing suit season.

Calorie Tracking Made Easy

Now that you know the parts played by calories, metabolism, and energy balance in losing fat tissue, what are your best next steps?

If you really want to lose fat tissue, I hope you are beginning to see the benefits of tracking what you eat with an App like MyFitnessPal. Even though tracking calories is a universally unpopular idea, you'll learn that it's a small price to pay for the control it offers you over your progress. Here's how it will help you.

You'll see first-hand how what you eat directly affects your weight. The day after I eat too many tortilla chips at the Mexican restaurant, I know exactly how the scale will respond. How do I know? I've done it many times and tracked it many times. Seeing the result, I'm also more likely to avoid doing it.

Another benefit of tracking that's easy to miss is the "training" that's occurring right under your nose. The attention and repetition you practice in tracking your food are the actions that result in the "lifestyle change" so often touted as the key to success. Each day you log your food intake, you'll practice the awareness and attention needed to govern your food choices and how they affect your weight.

You'll learn that fluctuations are normal and predictable. Your weight will bounce its way down gradually if you are consistently establishing a calorie deficit. If your weight isn't on a slow, downward trend, you'll know it's time to examine your calories or the accuracy of your tracking.

You'll also learn how to balance your calories and food choices so that you still feel satisfied. This may be the biggest benefit of all – developing a way to eat that you enjoy, feel satisfied, but aren't overeating. That's when you can lose weight slowly and not feel like you are dieting. This is the key to controlling your long-term success.

The next time someone says that to lose weight, "you have to change your lifestyle," know this: They probably have no clue what that looks like, but you will. If you are tracking what you eat and adjusting accordingly, you are doing what it takes to change your lifestyle.

Some of my clients have become so good at knowing their eating routine that they only need to track food intake a few days a week to stay in check. Personally, I still track my food and calories every day. It's a form of accountability I need – but I also enjoy. I know myself. It's too easy for me to eat too much without realizing it. I also like being in the driver's seat when it comes to my weight and my health.

I recommend tracking daily to stay accountable to your body's God-given calorie limit. Eating within your limit will remind you that your body is His, not yours.

Here's a summary of the rewards you'll enjoy by logging your food intake:

- It keeps you mindful of your daily limit, which helps prevent overeating.

- It ensures you are making progress toward your goal.

- You'll have a history of food choices to review and adjust. You won't have to wonder, "What am I doing wrong?"

- It gives you the freedom to build your own healthy eating plan rather than follow someone else's diet.

- It puts the power to lose fat tissue right in your hands.

In my experience, tracking calories is *the* best practical tool to lose fat tissue. It teaches you to honor the limits built into your body by God. He gave you a metabolism, and with it, a boundary limiting how much energy your body needs.

Those who track food intake consistently will end up with the most success in losing weight and keeping it off. The alternative of not tracking sets you up to flounder, get discouraged, and become stuck in a pattern of trying but not getting anywhere.

Do you want to know for sure that the effort you are making to lose weight is working? If so, then make an app like MyFitnessPal part of your daily routine.

Reflections

All the practical tools you need to manage your weight are simple and free. Practical tools are part of the picture. It's one thing to know about these tools and another thing to use them. I haven't met anyone who was genuinely excited about doing it at first. My recommendation is to start by downloading a tracking app and learning how it works. Take one step, regardless of how small, each day.

There were some difficult steps I needed to take. But they became easier when I decided I wanted to honor God in my body and choices. That was different than trying to fight hand-to-hand combat against my desires and cravings. God was equipping me to do what He was calling me to do: to leave my bondage behind.

Are you encouraged by the call to be a good steward of your body, God's temple? Even if you feel apprehensive about what it might entail, keep taking your anxious thoughts and feelings to God in prayer. Ask God to show you your heart clearly and to help you find a path to stewardship that pleases Him.

Questions
Read Colossians 1:10-12.

...so as to walk in a manner worthy of the Lord, fully pleasing to him: bearing fruit in every good work and increasing in the knowledge of God; [11] *being strengthened with all power, according to his glorious might, for all endurance and patience with joy;* [12] *giving thanks to the*

Father, who has qualified you to share in the inheritance of the saints in light.

1. How does being a good steward of your body relate to "walking in a manner worthy?"

2. Is it possible to lose weight but not walk in a manner worthy? What might be an example?

3. Has losing weight ever been a higher priority in your mind than increasing in the knowledge of God? It certainly has for me. Reflect on where your heart is now.

4. How can you increase in the knowledge of God?

5. Write out a prayer expressing where you are in being a good steward of your body. Ask for His help with the changes you see you may need to make.

Read Galatians 6:7-9.

Do not be deceived: God is not mocked, for whatever one sows, that will he also reap. ⁸ For the one who sows to his own flesh will from the flesh reap corruption, but the one who sows to the Spirit will from the Spirit reap eternal life. ⁹ And let us not grow weary of doing good, for in due season we will reap, if we do not give up.

6. Based on these verses, what consequences can we expect for our actions? What consequences are you experiencing now from the choices you've been making for your body?

7. What changes would you like to make now and over time?

8. How do these verses exhort you to keep going, even if you stumble?

Chapter Four:
What Should I Eat? (and why it's a useless question)

When you think about losing weight, what's the first thing that comes to your mind? For me, it was always this question: What *could* I eat? The next was "What would I have to *stop* eating?"

During my dieting decades, I logged my fair share of hours in the "Diet and Weight Loss" section of the bookstore. Every time I looked at a new diet book, I went straight to the part that told me what foods were "in" and which ones were "out." Before I purchased the book or started the diet, I was already figuring out ways to blur the lines. If I was going to do another stupid diet, I was going to do it *my* way, which, of course, never worked.

Most who have struggled to lose weight already know what we *should* eat. The problem is we don't want to eat what we ought to, nor stop eating what we prefer. I always held out hope that I could find a forgiving "diet" menu that allowed *plenty of* fried chicken and key lime pie.

Apart from illness or fasting, feeding ourselves has been a daily occurrence from the first time we pushed a toddler-sized fistful of Cheerios into our tiny baby pie holes. For all the days of your life, you have reinforced your deeply rooted and deeply personal point of view about eating and food. This mostly unconscious point of view is like an operating system, working in the background, guiding the decisions we make every day.

If you prepare food for others, your point of view infiltrates their lives as well. What has shaped your current eating philosophy? For me, the shaping hand of my family is apparent. Also, the American culture and period I grew up in—the tail end of the baby boom—is imprinted upon me as well. No doubt, our culture today plays a significant role in our beliefs about food as well as our decisions and preferences.

The subject of this chapter, "What should I eat?" is a potentially complicated question. The more people you ask, the more complicated it seems. Even some of the good answers seem to conflict. Surprisingly, the Bible is a simple place to start to determine what to eat. Granted, what to eat is more straightforward than making ourselves eat what we ought. The practice of following through on what we should eat will be discussed in greater detail in Part 3. First things first: the "what."

Take Me to Your Refrigerator

Imagine you are an alien sent to earth to study American eating behavior. What would you conclude that Americans believe about food?

Compare your answer to this 2012 study[16] that discovered that Americans decide what to eat based on this order of priority:

- Taste – 87%
- Price – 73%
- Healthfulness – 61%
- Convenience – 53%
- Sustainability (environmental impact) – 35%

The study also said, "While Americans acknowledge room to improve and report they are trying to improve the healthfulness of their diet, over half (54%) report that they would rather just enjoy their food than worry too much about what's in it."

Even so, a May 22, 2015 article in *Fortune Magazine* estimated that financial spending in the weight loss industry was $66 Billion in 2017.[17]

Now, recall the low success rates of diet programs. We spend billions of dollars on products that result in dismal weight loss success rates. Why do we keep buying products that have never been proven to work?

The purveyors of weight loss programs know us well. We want to enjoy our food, but we'd also really like to lose weight. Their answer? Diet products that give us what we want in the food—great taste, low price, fast weight loss, and convenience. We get all this but not the outcome we seek: permanent weight loss.

Diet programs sell the *hope* of losing weight without disrupting your life. Unfortunately, the advertising works far better than the programs. There's no evidence of any progress to stem the tide of Americans growing larger.

We spend $66 billion on products that fail 95% of the time. If two-thirds of Americans are overweight or obese, and 95% of weight loss efforts fail, we aren't talking about a small segment of struggling people. We are talking about *most* people. Now, think about the question at hand: "What should I eat?" Of all the proposed answers about what to eat, not one of the answers has been able to resolve this growing problem.

So, I must ask, what good is the question, "What should I eat?"

"You should eat vegetables," some will answer. Does that help? Not really. Not enough.

Among the problems with this question is its lack of specificity. Is "What should I eat to lose weight?" any better? Considering the Twinkie Diet resulted in weight loss, I'm still not satisfied with the helpfulness of the question.

"What should I eat to lose weight and be well-nourished?" Well, choose one of many healthy diets: Mediterranean, the DASH Diet, Weight Watchers, and others that you've tried. All of these could be nourishing and result in initial weight loss. But have any of the healthy diets you've been on before resulted in permanent weight loss?

Any version of the question, "What should I eat?" presumes there must be a way to eat that would result in permanent weight loss. But what if most people can't or simply won't eat that way? That seems to be where we now are in this culture. We have more nutrition information than ever, more diet programs than ever, and an obesity epidemic on the rise.

So, I propose two separate questions:

1) For now, what food does your body need to be nourished to reach and sustain a healthy weight?

2) For later, how does a person replace deeply embedded routines and preferences with new routines and preferences?

Recently, my pastor used a helpful illustration. He discussed the difference between Jesus using the words "go" and "come." When Jesus says "come," He is referring to a single destination: Himself. When He says the word "go," He could mean unlimited destinations. You can come to one place to start—with the truth. Then, when you have the truth, you can take it with you everywhere.

Let's start with the truth about what your body is designed to eat.

Born This Way

The eating philosophy woven into us day by day in life is powered by another internal drive: we want frequent and immediate gratification. It is so "normal," we scarcely realize it's there. The tendency to overeat and gain weight is the routine work of our flesh nature.

Most of the time, we don't think about God's intentions for food and eating. How does our philosophy about food and eating compare to God's truth about food and eating?

When God made us, He gave us the need to eat. He designed food to satisfy and sustain the human body. God's intention for food and eating are revealed in His Word. Considering our fallen nature, it's not surprising that our perspective has strayed from His perspective.

God created food *for us*, for our good. He provides us survival, enjoyment, nourishment, strength, and health so that we can walk with Him and fulfill the purpose He has for us. He made eating pleasurable. He gave us internal signals that tell us when we need to eat and when we've had enough.

After the Fall, when everything changed, our relationship with food was part of that change. God told Adam that mankind would have to work to produce food and that his labor would be painful. (See Genesis

3:17.) From that time until now, laboring for food has consumed most of our time and effort. Even if you aren't a farmer or a hunter, modern food production is still laborious. We may not grow or kill the food on our tables, but why do we work? So that we can afford to feed our families. We still labor for food. Given that we need food to survive, we are locked into the requirement to procure it.

Consider the "source material" of all foods, nature. Consider also mankind's ultimate lack of control over nature. Floods, droughts, weather patterns, and all kinds of elements beyond our control keep us dependent on God, whether we acknowledge it or not. Today, it's easy to lose sight of our ultimate dependence on God for food. When we forget, we are at risk of being arrogant and ungrateful. The earth is His and all it contains (Psalm 24:1). If there was ever a good reason to seek the Lord for guidance about food and eating, this is it. We must remember who we are in relation to Him.

God made food that is perfectly designed for our bodies. So, what does God think we should eat? That's actually a very good question, if I do say so myself.

A New Philosophy

To adopt a new way of thinking about food and eating, we must ask four questions:

- What does God's design teach us?

- What does God intend for us to eat?

- How does God intend for us to eat from day to day?

- What do we know about how God wants us to relate to food?

None of the diet books I read answered any of these questions. I hadn't asked these questions before. These are not diet-questions; they are relationship questions. At first, I didn't want to ask them, fearing the answers could be downright dreadful. What if God never wanted me to taste another white chocolate macadamia nut cookie? Whatever the case, I needed to know because He is my God, and this was an area where He was pressing on me to pay attention.

What Does God's Design Teach Us?

God's design teaches us. Much of what we need to know is built into us. The way our bodies tell us we need food and how our bodies respond to food came from God's creative mind. It's no surprise that our bodies respond well to healthy food and sensible exercise. We know we need daily nourishment and care for long-term maintenance. The demands of our bodies prove we are dependent on God. Our survival depends on how we attend to the needs our bodies present.

What Does God Intend for Us to Eat?

God's food occurs in nature, not in a lab or in a processing facility. This makes knowing what to eat simple. If God made it for food, and if man has not processed it, re-engineered it, or made a science project out of it, then it's good for food.

Most people don't eat this way, nor do they want to. A woman in one of my classes commented that if she opened her refrigerator and saw only fruits, vegetables, and whole foods, she would conclude that there was "nothing there to eat" and would order a pizza. What God intended for us to eat is relatively straightforward. Even though the "how" is a real challenge, the "what" is not nearly the mystery we have made it out to be.

How Does God Intend for Us to Eat from Day to Day?

It's good news that The Bible and our bodies tell us more than we may realize about how to eat. Practically speaking, we mainly need to know two things: what to eat and how much. We know that God made a variety of plant-based foods for Adam and Eve to eat (Genesis 1:29-30). He told Noah and his family that in addition to the vegetation, the animals that roamed the earth would be food for them. God also made animals afraid of us, so He apparently intended for us to chase them (Genesis

9:2-3). Whether it was the main purpose, I can't say, but God's design requires that we exert ourselves to obtain food from the earth.

Today, the nature of the effort is different. We work to pay for food, but we expend very little effort or energy to obtain it. The unforeseen consequence of man's progress is often his own demise.

Not surprisingly, our bodies respond well to the food He designed for us, and they respond poorly to processed food and overeating. God has built into our bodies physiological disincentives for our poor decisions. Weight gain and weight-related illnesses are indications we are straying outside the natural boundaries God set in the design of our bodies.

Finally, our bodies tell us how much to eat. As we discussed in an earlier chapter, God gave each of us a metabolic limit. He also gave us a complex internal signaling system that alerts us to hunger, thirst, satisfaction, and pleasure. The problem is that we ignore the subtle stop signals in favor of the much louder pleasure signals that distort our relationship to food.

How Does God Want Us to Relate to Rood?

God wired instincts and intrinsic rewards into our nature for our survival. He made eating pleasurable. Like all the pleasurable and beautiful things He created, they can be a blessing or a snare.

In Deuteronomy 8:3, Moses reminds the Israelites. "And He humbled you and let you hunger and fed you with manna, which you did not know, nor did your fathers know, that He might make you know that man does not live by bread alone, but man lives by every word that comes from the mouth of the Lord."

God gave them very specific instructions about the manna. He told them how to gather it, when to gather it, and how much to gather. He was testing them. Would they obey His instructions? Would they recognize what He was teaching them? Would they learn to depend on Him?

They were being fed something He had provided uniquely for them to demonstrate that He was their God and that they were His people, unlike any other nation on the earth. Would they respond appropriately to this unique Divine relationship, being fully cared for and loved by God Almighty?

Just as it did for Israelites, food can expose our hearts. How did they do with the Lord's test? They complained. "We remember the fish we ate in Egypt that cost nothing, the cucumbers, the melons, the leeks, the onions, and the garlic. But now our strength is dried up, and there is nothing at all but this manna to look at" (Numbers 11: 5-6). Of course, God could hear them.

After all God had done and was doing for them, they were fantasizing about the food back in Egypt. Why couldn't they see the big picture?

Has God done any less for us today? We've seen more of God's work than the Israelites saw. We've seen God's promises to them fulfilled in Christ. Is God any less interested in the way we relate to food? Even today, our need for food and our ability to obtain food depends on Him. Our circumstances make it easy to forget. Yet in forgetting, we show the same disdain for God and His overwhelming generosity that the Israelites did.

All of God's gifts, including food and eating, teach us about Him. But God never meant for food to master us or to become our longing, comfort, entertainment, or a source of constant self-gratifying pleasure. It was intended to point us to Someone greater than the gift—to the Giver of all gifts.

Food has become a tool and a snare that the enemy uses to stir up our flesh and direct our attention to ourselves. In Part 3, we'll explore our vulnerability to our flesh nature and how the enemy of our souls tempts us with food to weaken and undermine us spiritually.

In our food-worshipping culture, how does a person who wants to honor God find her or his way back to a God-honoring relationship with food?

Practically speaking, we can take what God reveals in His Word and develop guidelines to eating in a God-honoring way. Some commonly used nutrition concepts will help connect God's guidelines with the practical boundaries we can set for ourselves.

Nutrition: What Do Our Bodies Need to Function Properly?

Having established that God made the foods we are designed to eat, we can rejoice that He offers us an abundance of choices. Our bodies need a variety of nutrients, and we are naturally attracted to a variety of foods. To help you shape a plan that includes the variety of nutrients your body needs most, let's review these basic nutrition concepts: macronutrients and micronutrients. These will help us learn the language of better informed food decisions.

What is a Macronutrient and Why Does it Matter?

Look at any food's nutrition label, and you will see a breakdown of the calories into protein, fat, and carbohydrate grams, along with many other details. The three categories—protein, fat, and carbohydrates—are known as macronutrients. Yes, this is common knowledge. But less commonly known are what "macronutrient" means and how each of the three differs from the others.

Macronutrients are so named because our bodies require them in larger quantities than their petite cousins, the micronutrients, which we'll also touch on.

Why do macronutrients matter? Because they behave differently from each other in your body.

The National Institute of Health recommends that we structure our eating so that we get our total calories in these macronutrient proportions:[18]

Macronutrient	Recommended range
Carbohydrate	45% to 65%
Fat	20% to 35%
Protein	10% to 35%

The proposed ranges offer flexibility while ensuring your body has enough of each. What qualifies a food to fall into its respective category?

If you were to look at *one molecule* of each macronutrient, you would see three different structures. The chemical elements comprising them and how the elements are bonded or connected to each other are different. You may not care, but your body notices. Rather than balance a few chemical equations (as if I could), consider this metaphor as a more relatable illustration.

Recall the children's story The Three Little Pigs. Imagine each macronutrient is one of the three types of materials to build the little pigs' houses. One is made of sticks, one of wood, and one of bricks. Just as the construction of the pigs' houses determined how easily they were broken down by the wolf's huffing and puffing, each macronutrient breaks down differently, and some more easily than others.

One gram of protein and one gram of carbohydrate each have four calories. But your body treats proteins and carbs differently because of their different molecular structures. A carbohydrate is more like the pig's stick house, the easiest to break down. The protein is more like the second pig's house, which was made of wood and takes a little more huffing and puffing. As a result, your body makes use of them differently: carbohydrates to fuel activity, and protein more for repair and building tissue.

Now, consider one gram of fat. One gram of fat, the same size volume-wise, is denser. It has more than double the energy: nine calories. It's the brick house in our "three little pigs" analogy. Its greater calorie density isn't necessarily a bad thing. Our bodies need dietary fat for many reasons, including cellular level functions, which extend far beyond my ability to describe.[19] The fat calories you eat behave differently from protein and carbs. The point is our bodies need all three types of macronutrients in varying amounts, and they perform varying functions.

Calorie Inequality is Really Nutritional Inequality

When people say that "not all calories are created equal," this is what they are getting at: Proteins, carbohydrates, and fats differ structurally and so, behave differently in your body. Nutritionally speaking, 100 calories of peanut butter is different than 100 calories of cauliflower, even though they are equal in energy.

But not only do macronutrients differ from each other, but there are important differences within each category that matter when it comes to our health. There are subtypes of each macronutrient that are worse for us because of their structure. For instance, the carbohydrates that are easiest to break down are typically worse for our bodies than others.

Subtypes such as simple vs. complex carbohydrates, saturated vs. unsaturated fats, and animal vs. plant proteins, are structural differences your body notices. Ergo, it would be *unwise* to construct a diet out of pretzels, cake frosting, and spam, even if you could achieve a "healthy" macronutrient balance.

The problem with a pretzel-frosting-spam diet or the variations of equally unhealthy typical American diets is that such diets are devoid of micronutrients. What are micronutrients?

What is a Micronutrient?

Micronutrients are the vitamins and minerals found in food and dietary supplements. They are called micronutrients because they are substances our bodies require in minuscule quantities. For instance, my body needs the micronutrient magnesium in the recommended daily amount of 0.32 grams, whereas I need about 175 grams total of the macronutrient carbohydrate.

Our bodies need a wide variety of these tiny micronutrients. How can you be sure your body is getting what it needs? Not surprisingly, the foods God made, in their most natural forms, are the richest sources of micronutrients. By eating vegetables, fruits, grains (non-genetically modified), some nuts and seeds, some forms of animal protein, and beans, we can get most if not all the micronutrients we need. Micronutrients from real food are the best sources for your body.

If asking "What should I eat?" is the wrong question, what is a better question? Asking the question "What has God revealed that this body He designed needs?" is a great place to start. This will help you build an eating plan that will give your body what it needs as well as how much it needs. Here are a few suggestions:

1. Learn what your personal calorie limit is and practice staying within range. When you create a consistent calorie deficit, you will achieve slow and steady weight loss.

2. Identify the "God-made" foods you like and incorporate more of them into your diet. A resource I have found helpful is *The World's*

Healthiest Foods website. Their list of the 100 Healthiest Foods provides a great list to build from.

3. Progressively reduce processed foods and fast foods from your daily and weekly routine. The more processed foods you can eliminate over time, the better.

4. Educate yourself about food quality. There are many documentaries that will teach you how to choose "cleaner" foods.

5. Keep a standard grocery list that you tweak and improve over time.

6. Don't aim for perfection; it is an insatiable master. Be patient and give yourself grace when you stumble. Everyone does.

7. Expect to stumble.

8. Expect to recover from every stumble. Develop a recovery routine. In the diet world, a stumble can mean the end. When you are honoring God in your body, you get up and keep going. After you have recovered a few times, you realize it's not as hard as you thought to get back on track.

9. Make a tracking app like MyFitnessPal a part of your routine. It may seem tedious at first, but it is like having a GPS to guide you to your destination.

Transitioning from eating an American diet to eating by God's design takes time. While it may not be as fast, easy, or convenient as you'd like, neither is dieting. But eating God's way is a deeply meaningful and worthwhile pursuit when the aim is something so exceedingly worthy—pleasing God and escaping the enslaving power of processed food.

As with all new things, it will get easier and even more enjoyable as you grow in strength and skill. The new routines you work on little by little will become your new habits. With consistency, your new routine will become your new normal, and the hardest part of the shift will be behind you.

Reflections

The changes I made that finally stuck with me were neither sudden nor drastic. The more prayerfully and thoughtfully I approached the changes, the more real and sustainable my progress was. I transitioned away from the stop and start of yo-yo dieting and enjoyed my new relationship with food.

When I asked, "What would it look like to honor God in the way I ate, drank and lived?" I knew part of the answer was that my relationships had to change, both with food and with God.

I encourage you to take a thoughtful and prayerful approach to the changes you will make and that God will make in you. Allow Him to speak to your heart about His desire for the care of your body, the temple He calls His dwelling place.

Questions
Read Daniel 1:8-9.

But Daniel resolved that he would not defile himself with the king's food, or with the wine that he drank. Therefore he asked the chief of the eunuchs to allow him not to defile himself. ⁹ And God gave Daniel favor and compassion in the sight of the chief of the eunuchs,

1. Daniel, a young Jewish man, was raised under specific dietary laws given by God to the Israelites. Why do you think it was important to Daniel not to defile himself while he was in captivity under the Babylonians?

2. When God looked on Daniel's heart, what do you think He saw?

Read 2 Corinthians 7:1.

Since we have these promises, beloved, let us cleanse ourselves from every defilement of body and spirit, bringing holiness to completion in the fear of God.

3. We are not under the specific dietary restrictions that God gave the Israelites, but is God is concerned with how you treat your body today? Describe ways a person might displease the Lord as it relates to eating.

4. How might a person's eating or their relationship with food represent a "defilement?"

5. What could a person do to pursue holiness in how he/she eats?

Read Matthew 6: 31-33,

Therefore do not be anxious, saying, 'What shall we eat?' or 'What shall we drink?' or 'What shall we wear?' ³² For the Gentiles seek after all these things, and your heavenly Father knows that you need them all. ³³ But seek first the kingdom of God and his righteousness, and all these things will be added to you.

6. Is it possible to become overly concerned with your body, or what you eat?

7. In what ways does anxiousness about other things affect your eating habits?

8. What does it mean to "seek first the kingdom of God?" Answer to the best of your ability. But also, ask the Lord to reveal to you what He meant when He said it, and how to make it an ever-increasing reality in your life.

Chapter Five:
Exercise?

Have you ever watched a sporting event and felt inspired to get in shape? Certain sports inspire me more than others; tennis, track and field, and soccer are my specific motivators. After watching Wimbledon each year, I felt inspired to hit the gym, the tennis courts, and buy new running shoes. Shortly thereafter, the shine faded back into reality.

The work was hard, and my body was downright uncooperative. It refused to morph into what I envisioned: a sleek, sculpted form resembling those athletes who made it look so easy.

When I was younger, I was willing to put in the time. I'm pretty sure I was an exercise bulimic before it had a name. However, the four hours or so I channeled into exercise each day never made enough of a dent in my subcutaneous fat to reveal a sculpted and toned physique, if it was even in there somewhere.

Does exercise really help with weight loss? What if the answer is "no," or "not all that much?"

Make no mistake; exercise is beneficial to our bodies. But how much does exercise really influence weight loss? In this chapter, I simply want to clarify what exercise will and won't do when it comes to losing weight. It's also worth asking, "How much exercise do our bodies really need?"

Where Possibility Meets Practicality

I learned the limitations of exercise the hard way. While I was so determined to exercise my way thin, I was making big errors in judgment:

1) I thought I could out-exercise what I was eating.

2) I assumed the people with those enviable bodies achieved them with exercise and never worried about what they ate.

I was determined to earn my freedom to eat whatever I wanted. Addressing what I ate was off the negotiating table. I would do anything *but* expose what I ate to potential curtailment.

Now, it's easier for me to see this in hindsight. Back then, I was too close to it to recognize what I was doing.

Right-Size Your Expectations

When I hear someone say that they need to start exercising *because* they think it will help them lose weight, my antenna twitches. Whether it's fair or not, I suspect one of two things: either they mistakenly believe the widespread myth that exercise leads to weight loss or, like me, they consider jogging or Zumba (or whatever) lesser evils when compared to giving up peanut M&Ms and other food freedoms.

Where does exercise lose its punch in weight loss? Answer: It is no match in calorie burning for its most powerful opponent, eating and calorie accumulating. Case in point: A person can eat 1,000 calories in 10 minutes. It takes two hours or more to burn them off.

The calories we eat tally up far faster than the calories we burn. Think about it. Mankind wouldn't have survived before industrialization if a little food didn't go a long way. Eating used to involve a whole lot more running around to put a much smaller yield of calories on the "table." Today, we can have French toast and bacon from fridge to table in less than 30 minutes. This has only been possible for a tiny sliver of human history. The human body was made to survive in high-calorie expenditure and calorie-scarcity. We live in calorie-abundance and low-expenditure. Our environment has changed drastically. The needs of our bodies have not.

To complicate matters for us modern folks, most of us far *overestimate* the calories we burn during exercise and far *underestimate* how many calories we eat. This is the perfect storm for the most frustrating kind of weight gain: the kind that occurs while you think you are trying hard.

Where weight loss (fat tissue loss) is concerned, studies have shown that exercise is no more beneficial than cutting calories. [20] Since the cause-and-effect relationship of exercise to weight loss is far weaker than most realize, it is worth rethinking the role exercise plays in one's weight loss journey and overall health. In other words, don't bank on exercising your way to weight loss, especially if you aren't paying attention to calories.

Then, Why Bother?

If exercise only minimally helps to lose weight, must you exercise at all? Yes. Our bodies need to move to be healthy. If you aren't already active, you might want to consider gradually developing a more active lifestyle – for your long-term health.

Of course, you must first ask your doctor, especially if you are at risk or being treated for any illness. Your physician is aware of any risks to your health imposed by your medical history, and he or she should be given the opportunity to give you an opinion.

Made to Move (Sitting Ourselves to Death)

God created our bodies to move. We are designed to walk between five and ten miles a day. Walking that far was easier to achieve before the days of wheeled and motorized transportation. Just as we aren't adapted for a calorie-intense environment, we aren't built for prolonged sitting around, which is common in modern cultures. Our bodies need to move, regardless of how infrequently our lives require it or how strongly we might resist it. In fact, not only our bodies but our brains function at their best when blood is pumping as the result of physical effort.[20]

A widely circulated study showed that sitting for extended periods of time is *worse* for us than smoking. In an interview with the *Los Angeles Times*, Dr. James Levine, director of the Mayo Clinic-Arizona State University Obesity Solutions Initiative, stated, "Sitting is more dangerous than smoking, kills more people than HIV and is more treacherous than parachuting. We are sitting ourselves to death." [21]

Dr. Levine originated the phrase "sitting is the new smoking." Many media outlets published articles on his research. *Runners World* highlighted the fact that *even if* you exercise for an hour a day, but the rest of the day you are sedentary, you are equally at risk for all the ill effects of sitting for prolonged periods of time. [22] That got my attention. Even considering the hour or so of cardio I did almost daily for my weight loss fantasy, I wasn't moving enough the rest of the day for my health.

Apart from the risks of being sedentary, what are the benefits of adopting a more active lifestyle? There are many.

Consider how many Americans suffer from weight-related illnesses, such as high blood pressure, heart disease, diabetes, and cancer. Exercise plays an important role in healing from these diseases. The body's ability to heal itself is built into us and enhanced by activity. You may know this from your own experience. Even so, the CDC lists the following documented benefits of physical activity:[23]

- Controls weight

- Reduces the risk of cardiovascular disease

- Reduces risk for type 2 diabetes and metabolic syndrome

- Reduces risk of some cancers

- Strengthens bones and muscles

- Improves mental health and mood

- Improves ability to do daily activities and prevent falls if you're an older adult

- Increases the chances of living longer

Exercise offers hope for better health to those who have slipped into any of the risks or diseases that go hand in hand with the underactive, overeating American lifestyle.

Does your body need the healing effects of exercise?

How to Start Increasing Activity

After your doctor gives you the green light, start slowly, especially if you aren't active. Choose an activity such as walking or a group exercise class that is geared toward your fitness level. Walking may become your main activity or one that supplements others. Either way, work toward reaching the minimum activity guidelines recommended by the Centers for Disease Control, or CDC. The official recommendation is 150 minutes of moderate activity per week, which would equate to 7,000-8,000 steps per day. [22]

Notice how many steps you take in a day. You can do this using a pedometer, a smartphone app, or a step-tracking device such as a Fitbit. Work toward increasing the number of steps you take each day little by little until you reach 8,000. You may wish to take it further. Many people aim for 10,000 steps. The origin of this guideline harkens back to the 1960s. Pedometers sold in Japan in the 1960s were marketed under the name "manpokei," which translates to "10,000 steps." [24] If walking is not possible for you, consider speaking with a physical therapist or personal trainer to help you find a safe way to move more.

Does your current daily routine involve a lot of sitting? Consider ways to add movement for a few minutes during each hour or so of the day. Apart from physical exercise, the amount of time you simply move around plays a significant role in your health and helps you burn a few more calories each day. Moving can make a more noticeable difference over time. I have a friend who owns a cleaning business. Her job requires her to burn far more calories in a day than my job, which involves sitting, typing, and talking. If you don't enjoy exercise, there are ways to get un-sedentary without specifically exercising.

N.E.A.T.

There is a name for the calories you burn from your daily activity that doesn't come from exercise. It is called non-exercise activity thermogenesis, or NEAT. Dr. James Levine, of the "sitting is the new smoking" fame, says that NEAT plays a significant role in explaining and managing obesity. [25]

One of the ways that I get more "N.E.A.T." in my sedentary job is by pacing while I'm on the phone, or taking five-minute walk breaks throughout my work day. I might pace while I watch TV or read while I walk up and down the hallway. Even if I only burn off an extra 100 calories per day with the extra moving around, the net difference is close to 10 pounds each year. That may be 10 pounds I don't gain, or it may help me lose a few, depending on how I manage what I eat.

Using my Fitbit tracking device motivates me to go a little further each day to reach my minimum goal. Small activities you perform consistently will work in ways that drastic and unsustainable measures never work.

Something simple you can do right now is this: set your alarm to get up and move around every hour or so. By doing this, you can counteract the adverse effects on your body of sitting and add to your N.E.A.T.-related calorie burn. Before you know it, your routine will include regular activity sufficient to improve your health.

N.E.A.T. and its impact on managing your health is good news for those who would rather have a tooth drilled than go to a gym or think about vigorous exercise. Some may find it reassuring to know that the gym is not the only place to start making strides toward better health.

Where weight loss (fat loss) is concerned, exercise is not as effective as most think at the beginning of your weight loss journey. Exercise's most powerful effect on weight comes in the phase of your journey when you are stabilizing and maintaining. This is another good reason to build it into your routine. It will help you maintain the weight you lose gradually as you make changes to what and how much you eat.

If you find you have ever fallen prey to the "exercise = more food mindset," you now have the tools to escape it. When you manage the calories you eat *and* burn, you'll be better equipped to control your health and your weight. Adding more activity to your daily routine will prepare you to sustain your weight loss.

Reflections

While much has been written on the topic of exercise, you can keep it simple by remaining mindful of God's design for your body and what you can realistically accomplish. Make sure the activities you choose match the ends you hope to achieve.

I hope these examples have equipped you to consider what goals are appropriate for you in exercise. Most of all, I hope you are encouraged to pursue asking the Lord to guide you and to give you a hunger to please Him in your pursuit of good bodily stewardship.

Questions

Read 1 Corinthians 9:24-27.

Do you not know that in a race all the runners run, but only one receives the prize? So run that you may obtain it. ²⁵ *Every athlete exercises self-control in all things. They do it to receive a perishable wreath, but we an imperishable.* ²⁶ *So I do not run aimlessly; I do not box as one beating the air.* ²⁷ *But* **I discipline my body and keep it under control***, lest after preaching to others I myself should be disqualified.*

1. What are some of the spiritual disciplines that are important to growing in maturity in your relationship with Christ?

2. How do physical disciplines that lead to better health relate to spiritual health?

Read Romans 8: 6-8.

For to set the mind on the flesh is death, but to set the mind on the Spirit is life and peace. ⁷ For the mind that is set on the flesh is hostile to God, for it does not submit to God's law; indeed, it cannot. ⁸ Those who are in the flesh cannot please God.

3. Is it possible to be spiritually healthy if your physical habits have more control over you than you have over them?

4. According to these verses, how does being anxious about food and body image deprive us of life and peace?

Read Romans 8: 9, 12-15.

You, however, are not in the flesh but in the Spirit, if in fact the Spirit of God dwells in you. Anyone who does not have the Spirit of Christ does not belong to him... So then, brothers, we are debtors, not to the flesh, to live according to the flesh. 13 For if you live according to the flesh you will die, but if by the Spirit you put to death the deeds of the body, you will live. 14 For all who are led by the Spirit of God are sons of God. 15 For you did not receive the spirit of slavery to fall back into fear, but you have received the Spirit of adoption as sons, by whom we cry, "Abba! Father!"

5. What does Paul mean when he says "by the Spirit put to death the deeds of the body"? How is this different than using your will power?

6. Describe the hope we have because we are in Christ.

Final Word

Have you ever looked back on a time of struggle in your life and seen it more clearly than you did while you were in the middle of it? Perhaps we all have. My weight was just one of those struggles. But it's the one where my emotions were the so-called friend who betrayed me at every turn. I can't imagine my feelings doing a better job of hindering me and keeping me stuck and miserable.

Emotions are tricky, to say the least. But they can be dismantled. In this book, I've walked you through the first part of the process. The process I proposed begins with getting grounded in truth, the truth about how God made our bodies.

Knowing the truth about how your body works in relation to losing fat accomplishes more than you may realize. Yes, you can take an approach to losing weight that reflects the way God made our bodies. But more than that, you can now begin to confront your emotions with this truth, standing on more solid ground.

There's no escaping the way God made us. Why would we want to? We are beautifully and wonderfully made. Aligning our lives with His design acknowledges we trust Him and desire to surrender ourselves to Him in every way.

I hope that you took the time to work through the questions at the end of each chapter. If you did, we began the process of confronting your emotions in preparation for the next step in the process.

After you have nailed down the truth about our bodies, the next step is to lean further into confronting our thoughts and emotions with more truth from God's Word.

With the foundation of truth about your body, you can stand firm as you continue to fight the battle. As my Pastor has said, in Christ, we fight *from* victory not *for* victory.

It's great news that the body God made for us works in predictable ways and that there are simple things we can do. Now, take full advantage of knowing the "what" so you can devote more attention to the long-term "how." God's Word and growth in Him will lead you to a changed relationship with food. His transforming work from the inside and your cooperation with Him will lead you to permanent weight loss. Be on the lookout for Part 3 in the *I Once Was Fat but Now I'm Found* series, which dives into God's work of transformation.

As I said in Part 1 of this series, losing weight permanently is much more than a physical or even psychological change. It requires the transforming work of Christ in our hearts. It is a spiritual change process that will unfold into changes in your choices, your relationship with food, and your health. These will be byproducts of the healing work the Lord wants to do in your life.

Ask the Lord to help you see your heart clearly and to give you the wisdom and willingness to move forward. Then, do your part to move forward with Him. When the Lord transforms our hearts, change becomes possible in a way we could never accomplish with mere willpower. Genuine change occurs only with God's power and our cooperation, and it needs to be reinforced within a community of believers.

There is more to come in the *I Once Was Fat* series. For more information about "Stop Dieting for Life" or our online course, check us out at StopDietingforLife.com

Notes

Chapter One

1. Berggren, Jason R., Matthew W. Hulver, and Joseph A. Houmard. "Fat as an Endocrine Organ: Influence of Exercise." Journal of Applied Physiology. 1 Aug. 2005: 757-64. Print.

2. Mercola.. January 2, 2009. *Fascinating Facts You Never Knew About the Human Brain.* http://articles.mercola.com/sites/articles/archive/2009/01/22/fascinating-facts-you-never-knew-about-the-human-brain.aspx

3. Fotuhi, Majid, MD, PhD; Brooke Lubinski. July/August 2013. *The Effects of Obesity on Brain Structure and Size.* http://practicalneurology.com/2013/08/the-effects-of-obesity-on-brain-structure-and-size

4. The Visual MD. (n.d.) Retrieved April 15, 2015. *Obesity* (Video). http://www.thevisualmd.com/health_centers/weighed_down_obesity/obesity/obesity_video

5. "What Are the Health Risks of Overweight and Obesity?" - NHLBI, NIH. Web. 22 June 2015.

6. Palmer, Nicole; Hassan W. Bakos; Tod Fullston; Michelle Lane. October 1, 2012. "Impact of obesity on male fertility, sperm function and molecular composition." http://www.ncbi.nlm.nih.gov/pmc/articles/PMC3521747/

7. Wikipedia. April 8, 2015. *Adipose Tissue.* http://en.wikipedia.org/wiki/Adipose_tissue

8. Berggren, Jason R., Matthew W. Hulver, and Joseph A. Houmard. "Fat as an Endocrine Organ: Influence of Exercise." Journal of Applied Physiology 1 Aug. 2005: 757-64. Print.

Chapter Two

9. "Calorie." Wikipedia: The Free Encyclopedia. Wikipedia Foundation, Inc., 22 June 2015. Web. 23 June 2015. https://en.wikipedia.org/?title=Calorie

10. Clarke DD, Sokoloff L. Regulation of Cerebral Metabolic Rate. In: Siegel GJ, Agranoff BW, Albers RW, et al., editors. Basic Neurochemistry: Molecular, Cellular and Medical Aspects. 6th edition. Philadelphia: Lippincott-Raven; 1999. Available from: http://www.ncbi.nlm.nih.gov/books/NBK28194/

11. Merritt, April. "RMR vs. BMR." ACE Fitness, 12 Apr. 2010. Web. 23 June 2015. http://www.acefitness.org/blog/616/bmr-versus-rmr

12. Fell, James. "The Myth of Ripped Muscles and Calorie Burns." The Los Angeles Times. 16 May 2011. Web. 23 June 2015. http://www.latimes.com/health/la-he-fitness-muscle-myth-20110516-story.html#page=1.

Chapter Three

13. Dansinger, MD, Michael L., Joi Augustin Gleason, MS, RD, John L. Griffith, PhD, Harry P. Selker, MD, and Ernst J. Schaefer, MD. "Comparison of the Atkins, Ornish, Weight Watchers, and Zone Diets for Weight Loss and Heart Disease Risk Reduction, A Randomized Trial." *JMAM* 293.No.1 (2005): 43-53. *Jamanetwrok.com*. American Medical Association. Web. 3 Mar. 2016.

14. Sacks, M.D., Frank, and George Bray, M.D. "Comparison of Weight-Loss Diets with Different Compositions of Fat, Protein, and Carbohydrates." *The New England Journal of Medicine* Vol 360.Issue 9 (2009). *NEJM.org*. Massachusetts Medical Society. Web. 13 July 2015. http://www.nejm.org/doi/pdf/10.1056/NEJMoa0804748

15. Kollias, Helen. "Case study: The Biggest Loser." Precision Nutrition. Accessed April 1, 2019. https://www.precisionnutrition.com/the-biggest-loser-study

Chapter Four

16. 2012 Food & Health Survey: Consumer Attitudes toward Food Safety, Nutrition and Health." Foodinsight.org. May 2, 2012. Accessed March 11, 2016. http://www.foodinsight.org/2012_Food_Health_Survey _Consumer_Attitudes_toward_Food_Safety_Nutrition_and_Health

17. https://www.prnewswire.com/news-releases/us-weight-loss-market-worth-66-billion-300573968.html

18. Manore, Melinda. "Exercise and the Institute of Medicine Recommendations for Nutrition." *PubMed.gov*, National Institute of Health, 4 Aug. 2005, www.ncbi.nlm.nih.gov/pubmed/16004827. Accessed 2015.

19. Grady, Denise. "Fat - The Secret Life of a Potent Cell." The New York Times 6 July 2004. Web. 22 June 2015. http://www.nytimes.com/2004/07/06/science/fat-the-secret-life-of-a-potent-cell.html

Chapter Five

20. Redman, Leanne M., Leonie K. Heilbronn, and Corby K. Martin, et.al. "Effect of Calorie Restriction with or without Exercise on Body Composition and Fat Distribution." *The Journal of Clinical Endocrinology & Metabolism* Vol 92.(3) (2007): Pp 865-772. Print.

21. Macvean, Mary. "'Get Up!' or Lose Hours of Your Life Every Day, Scientist Says." Latimes.com. The Los Angeles Times, 31 July 2014. Web. 18 July 2015. http://www.latimes.com/science/sciencenow/la-sci-sn-get-up-20140731-story.html

22. Yeager, Selene. "Sitting Is the New Smoking- Even for Runners." *Runnersworld.com*. Runners World, 20 July 2013. Web. 18 July 2015. http://www.runnersworld.com/health/sitting-is-the-new-smoking-even-for-runners

23. "The Benefits of Physical Activity." *Centers for Disease Control and Prevention*, Centers for Disease Control and Prevention, 13 Feb. 2018, www.cdc.gov/physicalactivity/basics/pa-health/index.htm#ReduceCardiovascularDisease

24. Rettner, Rachel. "The Truth About '10,000 Steps' a Day." *LiveScience.com*. Purch, 6 June 2015. Web. 18 July 2015. http://www.livescience.com/43956-walking-10000-steps-healthy.html (Return to text.)

25. Levine, M.D., PhD, James. "The "NEAT Defect" in Human Obesity: The Role of Nonexercise Activity Thermogenesis." Mayo Clinic Endocrinology Update Volume 2. Number 1 (2007): 1-2. Print.

About the Author

Laura Fulford is the founder and creator of **Stop Dieting for Life**™, a Christian weight loss program. A graduate of Wake Forest University (B.S. in Exercise Science), she works with groups and individuals, helping them abandon old food and weight strongholds and re-align with God's design for eating and living. The **Stop Dieting for Life**™ course is available online at stopdietingforlife.com.

TUNKHANNOCK PUBLIC LIBRARY
TUNKHANNOCK, PA 18657

J 7.25

JAIL 1.25

JAIL 4.25

Made in the USA
Columbia, SC
13 December 2019

I once was Fat, but now I'm found #2